TEENAGE TRIUMPH:

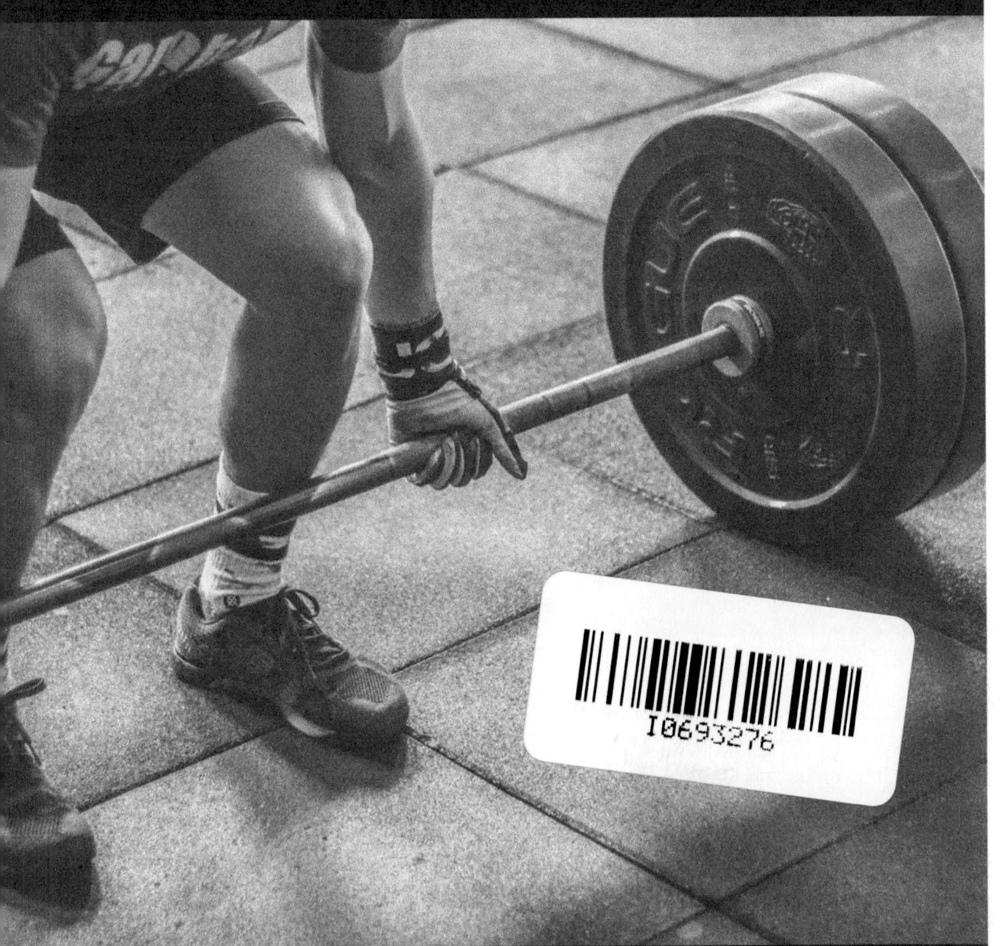

A FITNESS JOURNEY

by Eric L. Lloyd

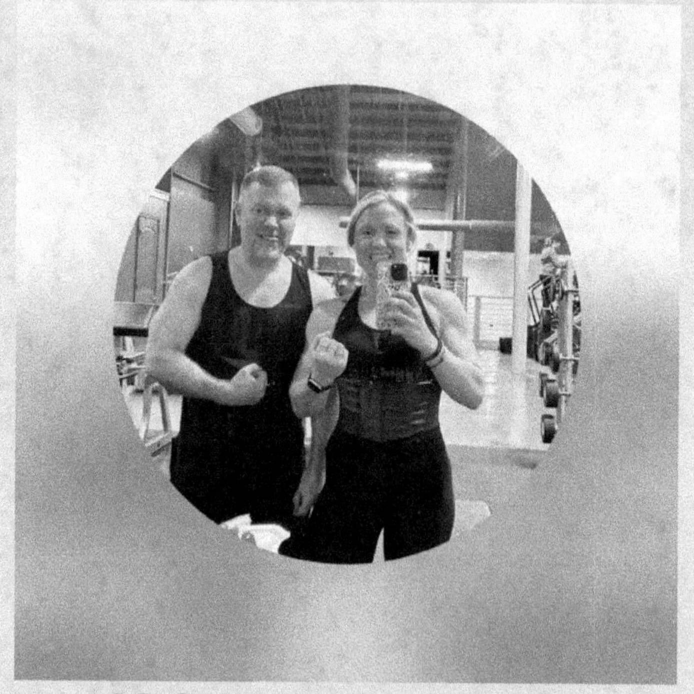

ABOUT THE AUTHOR

Born and raised in Dalton, GA, and currently living in Ringgold, GA, I have been working out since the eighth grade.....with a brief 4-5 year exception. That brief period of time is the inspiration behind this book. In this book, I hope to inspire many of you who may have had a similar fitness journey. I will share my experiences , education, and expertise in hopes that it will compel you to REVIVE & THRIVE!

Chapter 1: Setting the Stage

In the bustling halls of Heritage High School, a diverse tapestry of teenagers weaves its way through the maze of lockers and classrooms. Among them are our protagonists, each carrying their own burdens and aspirations, unaware of the journey that awaits them.

Meet Maya, a bookish introvert with a passion for art but struggling with body image issues that have plagued her since middle school. She navigates the halls with her head down, trying to blend into the background to avoid the judgmental stares of her peers.

Next is Alex, the star quarterback whose confidence on the field masks a deep insecurity about his physique. Despite his athletic prowess, he harbors doubts about his strength and endurance, especially as college scouts start to take notice.

Then there's Sophia, the class president and overachiever who juggles AP classes, extracurricular activities, and a part-time job with ease. But beneath her polished exterior lies a constant fear of failure and a desire to find balance in her hectic life.

Finally, we have Marcus, a shy musician who finds solace in his guitar but struggles to connect with others due to his social anxiety. He spends most of his free time holed up in his room, longing for a sense of belonging and purpose.

Despite their differences, Maya, Alex, Sophia, and Marcus share a common thread: a longing for change. They watch with a mixture of envy and curiosity as a group of students, led by a charismatic fitness enthusiast named Coach Ramirez, gather on the school's track every afternoon for intense workouts.

Coach Johnson is a legend at Heritage High, known for his passion for fitness and his ability to inspire others to push past their limits. His infectious energy and unwavering dedication to health and wellness have garnered him a cult-like following among students seeking to transform their bodies and minds.

.

As Maya, Alex, Sophia, and Marcus observe Coach Johnson and his disciples from a distance, a spark ignites within each of them. Maya yearns to feel confident in her own skin, Alex dreams of surpassing his physical limitations, Sophia seeks a reprieve from the relentless pressure to excel, and Marcus longs for the courage to step out of his comfort zone.

But the path to change is daunting, littered with obstacles and self-doubt. Maya worries that she'll never measure up to society's standards of beauty, Alex fears he'll never be strong enough to compete at the collegiate level, Sophia wonders if she'll ever find a way to silence the voice of doubt in her head, and Marcus questions whether he'll ever find the courage to break free from his self-imposed isolation.

As they stand on the precipice of transformation, Maya, Alex, Sophia, and Marcus must decide whether to take the first step toward a brighter future or remain mired in the familiar comforts of complacency. Little do they know, their lives are about to change in ways they never imagined, thanks to the power of fitness and the unwavering support of newfound friends.

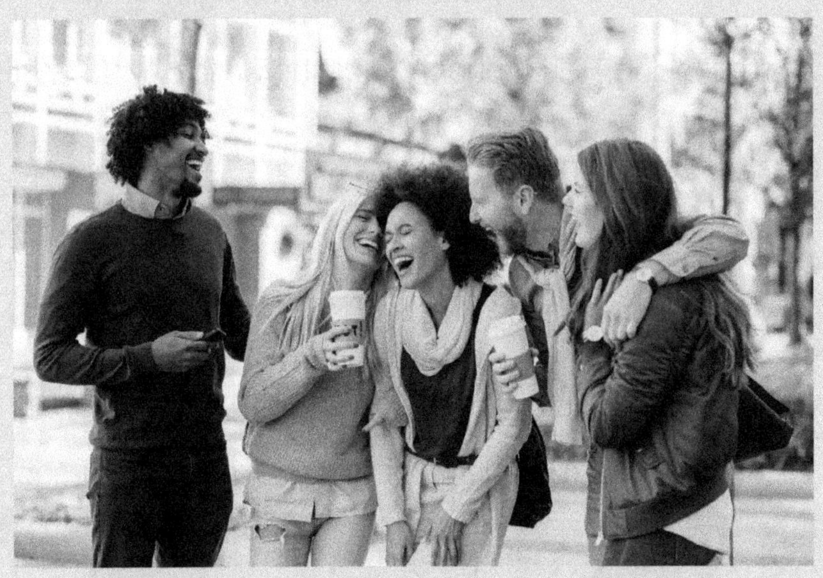

Chapter 2: The Spark of Inspiration

The sun dips low on the horizon, casting a warm glow over the school's track as Maya, Alex, Sophia, and Marcus linger nearby, watching Coach Johnson and his dedicated group of fitness enthusiasts. There's an energy in the air, a palpable sense of determination and camaraderie that draws them in like moths to a flame.

As Maya tentatively approaches the edge of the track, she feels a flutter of excitement mingled with apprehension. The thought of joining Coach Johnson's group fills her with both hope and trepidation. What if she's not fit enough? What if she embarrasses herself in front of everyone? But as she watches the sweat-drenched faces of the students pushing themselves to their limits, she can't help but feel a stirring of courage deep within her.

Alex stands a few feet away, his eyes fixed on Coach Johnson as he leads the group in a series of dynamic stretches. Despite his reservations, he can't deny the allure of the challenge laid out before him. He longs to test his limits, to prove to himself and others that he's capable of more than they realize. With a determined set to his jaw, he takes a step forward, ready to embrace whatever lies ahead.

Sophia hovers on the periphery, her mind a whirlwind of conflicting emotions. On one hand, she's drawn to the sense of community and purpose radiating from Coach Johnson's group. On the other hand, she worries about adding yet another commitment to her already overflowing plate. But as she watches the smiles of satisfaction and the high-fives exchanged between teammates, she can't help but feel a twinge of envy.

Maybe, just maybe, this is exactly what she needs to find balance in her hectic life.

Meanwhile, Marcus lingers in the shadows, his heart pounding with equal parts excitement and fear. The idea of stepping out of his comfort zone and joining Coach Johnson's group fills him with a sense of exhilaration unlike anything he's ever experienced. But the thought of drawing attention to himself, of being the center of attention, sends a shiver of anxiety down his spine. Can he muster the courage to take that first step into the unknown?

As the sun sinks lower in the sky, casting long shadows across the track, Maya, Alex, Sophia, and Marcus share a moment of silent solidarity. They may come from different backgrounds and face different challenges, but in this moment, they're united by a shared desire for change.

With a collective inhale, they take the plunge, stepping onto the track and into Coach Johnson's world of sweat, determination, and endless possibility. Little do they know, this single act of courage will set them on a path that will forever alter the course of their lives, igniting a spark of inspiration that will propel them forward on their journey to self-discovery and transformation.

Chapter 3: Overcoming Obstacles

The first day on the track with Coach Johnson is a baptism by fire for Maya, Alex, Sophia, and Marcus. As they join the group of dedicated students, they're immediately thrown into a whirlwind of high-intensity workouts and heart-pounding challenges. Sweat pours down their faces, muscles ache with exertion, and lungs burn with every labored breath. But amidst the physical discomfort, there's a sense of exhilaration unlike anything they've ever experienced.

For Maya, the biggest obstacle isn't the grueling workouts or the relentless pace—it's the voice of self-doubt that whispers in her ear with every step. As she struggles to keep up with the more experienced athletes, she can't help but compare herself to their toned bodies and effortless grace. But with Coach Johnson's encouragement and the support of her newfound friends, she pushes through the pain and embraces the challenge before her.

Alex, meanwhile, finds himself face to face with his own limitations. Despite his years of training on the football field, he quickly realizes that the demands of Coach Johnson's workouts are unlike anything he's ever encountered. Doubt creeps in as he struggles to keep pace with his peers, his muscles screaming in protest with each punishing rep. But with Coach Johnson's unwavering belief in his potential and the camaraderie of his fellow athletes, he digs deep and finds the strength to push past his perceived limitations.

Sophia grapples with a different set of obstacles as she tries to balance her newfound commitment to fitness with her already overflowing schedule. With AP classes, extracurricular activities, and a part-time job vying for her time and attention, she worries that she'll never find a way to make it all work. But as she immerses herself in Coach Johnson's workouts and connects with her fellow athletes, she discovers a newfound sense of focus and determination that helps her navigate the chaos of her busy life.

And then there's Marcus, whose battle with social anxiety threatens to derail his fledgling fitness journey before it even begins. As he steps onto the track with Coach Johnson's group, he feels the weight of a hundred eyes on him, judging his every move. But with each passing day, he finds solace in the supportive atmosphere of the group and the encouraging words of his newfound friends. Slowly but surely, he begins to shed the shackles of his self-imposed isolation and embrace the power of community.

As Maya, Alex, Sophia, and Marcus confront their individual obstacles head-on, they begin to realize that the path to self-improvement is paved with challenges and setbacks. But with determination, perseverance, and the unwavering support of Coach Johnson and their fellow athletes, they're ready to face whatever obstacles lie ahead. Little do they know, the trials and tribulations they encounter on the track will serve as the crucible that forges them into the strong, resilient individuals they're destined to become.

Chapter 4: Discovering Strengths and Weaknesses

As Maya, Alex, Sophia, and Marcus continue their journey with Coach Johnson's fitness group, they find themselves confronted with a myriad of physical and mental challenges. Each day brings new workouts, new obstacles to overcome, and new opportunities for self-discovery.

Maya, whose insecurities have long held her back, discovers a newfound sense of strength and resilience as she pushes herself to new limits on the track. Though she may not have the same level of athleticism as some of her peers, she quickly realizes that her determination and perseverance are her greatest assets. With each passing day, she finds herself growing stronger, both physically and mentally, as she learns to embrace her strengths and work on improving her weaknesses.

For Alex, the journey is one of self-discovery as he navigates the highs and lows of his athletic abilities. Though he may have once relied solely on his natural talent on the football field, he soon comes to understand that true strength comes from within. As he pushes himself through grueling workouts and tests his limits in ways he never thought possible, he discovers a newfound sense of pride in his abilities and a deeper appreciation for the power of hard work and dedication.

Sophia, too, finds herself grappling with her own strengths and weaknesses as she strives to balance her commitments on and off the track. Though she may excel in the classroom and in her extracurricular activities, she quickly learns that the demands of Coach Johnson's workouts require a different kind of skill set altogether. But with each passing day, she finds herself becoming more attuned to her body and its needs, learning to listen to its cues and push herself to new heights of physical fitness and endurance.

And then there's Marcus, whose journey of self-discovery takes on a whole new dimension as he confronts his social anxiety head-on. Though he may have once felt like an outsider on the track, he soon comes to realize that he's not alone in his struggles. As he connects with his fellow athletes and opens up about his fears and insecurities, he discovers a supportive community that accepts him for who he is. With each passing day, he finds himself growing more confident and self-assured, ready to take on whatever challenges lie ahead.

As Maya, Alex, Sophia, and Marcus continue to push themselves on the track, they begin to understand that true strength isn't just about physical prowess—it's about embracing your weaknesses, harnessing your strengths, and pushing yourself to be the best version of yourself possible. And with Coach Johnson and their fellow athletes by their side, they know that anything is possible.

Chapter 5: Building Resilience

As Maya, Alex, Sophia, and Marcus continue their fitness journey with Coach Johnson's group, they find themselves facing a series of setbacks and challenges that test their resolve and determination. But with each obstacle they encounter, they learn the importance of resilience—the ability to bounce back from adversity stronger than before.

For Maya, resilience takes on a whole new meaning as she grapples with injuries that threaten to derail her progress on the track. A strained muscle here, a twisted ankle there—it seems like every time she takes one step forward, she's forced to take two steps back. But rather than allowing herself to become discouraged, Maya uses these setbacks as an opportunity to reassess her approach and focus on other aspects of her fitness journey. With the help of Coach Johnson and her fellow athletes, she learns to listen to her body, take things slow, and adapt her workouts to accommodate her injuries.

And in doing so, she discovers a newfound sense of resilience that empowers her to keep pushing forward despite the obstacles in her path.

Meanwhile, Alex finds himself grappling with a different kind of setback as he struggles to balance his commitment to fitness with his responsibilities on the football field. With the start of the season looming on the horizon, he's torn between his desire to excel in both arenas and the fear that he may be spreading himself too thin. But rather than allowing himself to become overwhelmed, Alex chooses to lean into the challenge, using his time on the track as an opportunity to hone his skills and improve his endurance. And as he sees the progress he's making in his workouts translate onto the field, he gains a newfound sense of confidence in his abilities and a deeper appreciation for the power of resilience.

Sophia, too, finds herself facing her own set of challenges as she struggles to find balance in her hectic life. With AP exams, college applications, and a demanding part-time job all vying for her time and attention, she often finds herself feeling overwhelmed and exhausted. But rather than giving in to the pressure, Sophia chooses to prioritize her health and well-being, carving out time in her busy schedule for regular workouts with Coach Johnson and his group. And as she immerses herself in the world of fitness, she discovers a newfound sense of resilience that allows her to weather the storms of life with grace and determination.

And then there's Marcus, whose journey to resilience takes on a whole new dimension as he confronts the lingering effects of his social anxiety.

Though he may have made great strides in overcoming his fears on the track, he still finds himself grappling with moments of doubt and insecurity.

But rather than allowing himself to be consumed by fear, Marcus chooses to lean on the support of his fellow athletes and draw strength from their unwavering belief in his abilities.

As he faces each new challenge with courage and determination, he discovers a newfound sense of resilience that empowers him to embrace his true self and live life on his own terms.

As Maya, Alex, Sophia, and Marcus continue to navigate the ups and downs of their fitness journey, they come to understand that resilience isn't just about bouncing back from adversity—it's about embracing the challenges that come their way, learning from their experiences, and emerging stronger and more resilient than before. And with Coach Johnson and their fellow athletes by their side, they know that no matter what obstacles lie ahead, they have the strength and determination to overcome them.

Chapter 6: Finding Balance

As Maya, Alex, Sophia, and Marcus immerse themselves deeper into their fitness journey with Coach Johnson's group, they begin to realize the importance of finding balance in their lives. With the demands of school, extracurricular activities, and personal relationships pulling them in every direction, they discover that prioritizing their health and well-being is essential for achieving success both on and off the track.

Maya, who once struggled to find confidence in her own skin, finds solace in the rhythm of her workouts and the sense of accomplishment that comes with pushing her body to new limits. But as she throws herself wholeheartedly into her fitness journey, she quickly realizes that balance is key to maintaining her physical and emotional well-being. With Coach's guidance, she learns to listen to her body, prioritize rest and recovery, and find joy in activities outside of the gym. And in doing so, she discovers a newfound sense of equilibrium that allows her to thrive in all areas of her life.

For Alex, finding balance proves to be a delicate dance as he juggles his commitment to fitness with his responsibilities as a student-athlete. With the pressure to excel on the football field mounting with each passing day, he struggles to find time for workouts while still keeping up with his academic and social obligations. But rather than allowing himself to become overwhelmed, Alex chooses to embrace the challenge, using his time on the track as a form of stress relief and a means of sharpening his focus and discipline. And as he learns to prioritize his health and well-being, he discovers that true balance is not about dividing his time equally between competing demands, but rather about aligning his actions with his values and goals.

Sophia, too, finds herself grappling with the elusive concept of balance as she strives to excel in every aspect of her life. With the weight of expectations bearing down on her from all sides, she often feels as though she's teetering on the edge of burnout.

But rather than succumbing to the pressure, Sophia chooses to take a step back and reevaluate her priorities. With Coach Johnson's support, she learns to set boundaries, delegate tasks, and carve out time for self-care amidst the chaos of her busy schedule. And in doing so, she discovers a newfound sense of peace and fulfillment that allows her to thrive both academically and athletically.

And then there's Marcus, whose journey to finding balance takes on a whole new dimension as he confronts the lingering effects of his social anxiety. Though he may have made great strides in overcoming his fears on the track, he still finds himself struggling to connect with others outside of the gym. But rather than allowing himself to retreat into isolation, Marcus chooses to step outside of his comfort zone and embrace new opportunities for growth and connection. With Coach Johnson and his fellow athletes by his side, he learns to lean on others for support, seek out new experiences, and cultivate meaningful relationships that nourish his mind, body, and soul.

As Maya, Alex, Sophia, and Marcus continue to navigate the ups and downs of their fitness journey, they come to understand that finding balance is not a destination, but rather a continual process of self-discovery and self-care. And with Coach Johnson's guidance and the unwavering support of their fellow athletes, they know that no matter what challenges lie ahead, they have the strength and resilience to face them head-on and emerge stronger and more balanced than before.

Chapter 7: The Power of Community

As Maya, Alex, Sophia, and Marcus continue to push themselves on their fitness journey with Coach Johnson's group, they come to realize the transformative power of community. United by a shared commitment to health and wellness, they find strength, support, and inspiration in the bonds they form with their fellow athletes.

For Maya, who once felt isolated and alone in her struggles with body image and self-esteem, the sense of camaraderie she experiences on the track is nothing short of life-changing. Surrounded by teammates who lift her up and cheer her on, she feels a sense of belonging she's never known before. With each high-five, each word of encouragement, she feels her confidence grow and her fears fade away. And in the warm embrace of her newfound community, she discovers the courage to embrace her true self and live life on her own terms.

Similarly, Alex finds himself buoyed by the support of his fellow athletes as he navigates the challenges of balancing his commitments as a student-athlete. With their unwavering belief in his abilities and their willingness to push him to new heights, he feels a sense of motivation and determination unlike anything he's ever experienced. And as he crosses the finish line of each grueling workout, he knows that he couldn't have done it without the support of his teammates by his side.

Sophia, too, finds solace in the sense of connection she experiences with her fellow athletes as she struggles to find balance in her busy life. With their encouragement and understanding, she feels empowered to prioritize her health and well-being, even in the face of overwhelming pressure and expectations. And as she shares her triumphs and challenges with her teammates, she realizes that she's not alone in her struggles—that they're all in this together, supporting each other every step of the way.

And then there's Marcus, whose journey to overcoming social anxiety takes on a whole new dimension as he finds acceptance and belonging within Coach Johnson's group. With each new friend he makes and each connection he forges, he feels his fears and insecurities melt away, replaced by a sense of confidence and self-assurance he never thought possible. And as he embraces the power of community and opens himself up to the support of his fellow athletes, he knows that he'll never have to face life's challenges alone again.

As Maya, Alex, Sophia, and Marcus continue to grow and evolve on their fitness journey, they come to understand that true strength doesn't come from within—it comes from the connections we forge with others. In the warm embrace of their newfound community, they find the courage to push past their limits, the motivation to keep going when the going gets tough, and the inspiration to become the best versions of themselves possible..

And with Coach Johnson and their fellow athletes by their side, they know that no matter what challenges lie ahead, they'll always have a supportive community to lean on and lift them up.

Chapter 8: Facing Inner Demons

As Maya, Alex, Sophia, and Marcus continue their fitness journey, they find themselves confronted with a new set of challenges—this time, from within. Despite their physical progress and the unwavering support of their fellow athletes, they must grapple with their inner demons and confront the fears and insecurities that threaten to hold them back.

For Maya, the journey to self-acceptance is a rocky one, filled with moments of doubt and self-criticism. Despite her newfound confidence on the track, she still struggles to silence the voice of her inner critic—the one that tells her she's not good enough, not strong enough, not worthy of love and acceptance. But with each passing day, she learns to challenge these negative thoughts and replace them with words of kindness and self-compassion. With the support of her teammates and the guidance of Coach Johnson, she begins to see herself in a new light—as a strong, capable woman worthy of love and respect.

Similarly, Alex finds himself grappling with his own inner demons as he confronts the pressure to live up to the expectations placed upon him as a student-athlete. Despite his outward confidence and success on the field, he harbors doubts about his abilities and fears of failure that threaten to undermine his progress. But with the encouragement of his teammates and the wisdom of Coach Johnson, he learns to trust in himself and his abilities, recognizing that true strength comes not from perfection, but from resilience in the face of adversity.

Sophia, too, finds herself facing her own inner demons as she navigates the pressures of academic excellence and perfectionism. Despite her outward success and the admiration of her peers, she struggles with feelings of inadequacy and self-doubt that threaten to consume her. But with the support of her teammates and the guidance of Coach, she learns to let go of the need for perfection and embrace the beauty of imperfection.

And as she learns to accept herself for who she truly is, flaws and all, she discovers a newfound sense of freedom and joy that allows her to thrive in all areas of her life.

And then there's Marcus, whose battle with social anxiety continues to cast a shadow over his progress on the track. Despite his outward confidence and the acceptance of his teammates, he still struggles to silence the voice of his inner critic—the one that tells him he's not good enough, not worthy of love and acceptance. But with each passing day, he learns to challenge these negative thoughts and replace them with words of self-love and acceptance. With the support of his teammates and the guidance of Coach Johnson, he begins to see himself in a new light—as a valued member of the team, worthy of love and respect.

As Maya, Alex, Sophia, and Marcus continue to confront their inner demons and push past their fears and insecurities, they come to understand that true strength doesn't come from perfection, but from the courage to embrace their flaws and imperfections. And with the support of their teammates and the guidance of Coach Johnson, they know that they have the strength and resilience to overcome any obstacle that stands in their way.

Chapter 9: Celebrating Victories

As Maya, Alex, Sophia, and Marcus journey through their fitness transformation, they encounter numerous milestones, both big and small, that mark their progress and celebrate their victories. Each achievement, no matter how seemingly insignificant, serves as a testament to their dedication, resilience, and unwavering commitment to their fitness journey.

For Maya, the victories come in the form of small but significant triumphs over her insecurities and self-doubt. Whether it's completing a challenging workout without giving in to negative thoughts or noticing subtle changes in her body as she grows stronger and more confident, each accomplishment serves as a reminder of her inner strength and resilience. With each victory, Maya finds herself stepping more fully into her power, embracing her true self, and learning to love and accept herself unconditionally.

Similarly, Alex finds himself celebrating victories both on and off the field as he continues to push himself to new heights of athleticism and personal growth. Whether it's setting a new personal best in the weight room, leading his team to victory on the football field, or simply finding joy in the process of pushing his body to its limits, each achievement fills him with a sense of pride and accomplishment. With each victory, Alex gains a deeper appreciation for the power of perseverance and determination, knowing that no challenge is too great when approached with courage and tenacity.

Sophia, too, finds herself reveling in the victories that come with embracing imperfection and letting go of the need for perfection. Whether it's achieving a new personal best in her workouts, maintaining a healthy balance between her academic and personal life, or simply finding joy in the process of moving her body and nourishing her soul, each accomplishment serves as a reminder of her resilience and strength.

With each victory, Sophia learns to celebrate her progress rather than fixating on perfection, knowing that true happiness lies in embracing the journey rather than focusing solely on the destination.

And then there's Marcus, whose victories come in the form of newfound confidence and self-assurance as he continues to overcome his social anxiety and step into his power. Whether it's striking up a conversation with a teammate, speaking up in group settings, or simply feeling comfortable in his own skin, each achievement fills him with a sense of pride and accomplishment.

With each victory, Marcus gains a deeper appreciation for the power of vulnerability and authenticity, knowing that true connection and belonging come from embracing who he truly is rather than hiding behind a facade.

As Maya, Alex, Sophia, and Marcus celebrate their victories, they come to realize that true success isn't measured by external accolades or achievements, but by the growth and transformation that occurs within. Each victory, no matter how small, serves as a reminder of their strength, resilience, and unwavering commitment to their fitness journey. And with each triumph, they grow more confident, more resilient, and more empowered to face whatever challenges lie ahead.

Chapter 10: Embracing the Journey

As Maya, Alex, Sophia, and Marcus reflect on their fitness journey, they come to realize that the true beauty lies not in the destination, but in the journey itself. Each step, each struggle, and each triumph has shaped them into the strong, resilient individuals they are today, and they wouldn't trade a single moment of it for anything in the world.

For Maya, the journey has been one of self-discovery and empowerment. From overcoming her insecurities and self-doubt to embracing her strength and resilience, she has learned to love and accept herself unconditionally. Through the support of her teammates and the guidance of Coach Johnson, she has discovered a newfound sense of confidence and self-assurance that extends far beyond the track. And as she looks back on how far she's come, she knows that the journey is far from over—it's just beginning.

Similarly, Alex finds himself transformed by the journey, both physically and mentally. From pushing his body to new limits on the field to confronting his fears and insecurities head-on, he has grown stronger and more resilient with each passing day. Through the camaraderie of his teammates and the wisdom of Coach Johnson, he has learned to trust in himself and his abilities, knowing that true strength comes not from perfection, but from perseverance in the face of adversity. And as he looks ahead to the future, he knows that the lessons he's learned on the track will stay with him for a lifetime.

Sophia, too, finds herself forever changed by the journey. From learning to prioritize her health and well-being to embracing imperfection and finding balance in her busy life, she has discovered a newfound sense of peace and fulfillment that she never thought possible. Through the encouragement of her teammates and the guidance of Coach Johnson, she has learned to let go of the need for perfection and embrace the beauty of the journey, knowing that true happiness lies in embracing the process rather than fixating on the outcome.

And as she looks back on the obstacles she's overcome and the victories she's celebrated, she knows that the journey has been worth every step.

And then there's Marcus, whose journey to self-acceptance and belonging has been nothing short of transformative. From overcoming his social anxiety and finding connection with his fellow athletes to discovering the courage to be his authentic self, he has learned that true strength comes from vulnerability and authenticity. Through the support of his teammates and the guidance of Coach Ramirez, he has learned to embrace his true self and live life on his own terms, knowing that true happiness comes from embracing who he truly is rather than hiding behind a facade.

And as he looks ahead to the future, he knows that the journey has only just begun, and he's ready to face whatever challenges lie ahead with courage and conviction.

As Maya, Alex, Sophia, and Marcus stand together, united by their shared experiences and the bonds of friendship forged on the track, they know that the journey is far from over. But with each step they take, each obstacle they overcome, and each victory they celebrate, they grow stronger, more resilient, and more empowered to face whatever challenges lie ahead. And as they embrace the journey with open hearts and open minds, they know that the possibilities are endless, and the future is theirs for the taking.